I0421376

Fitbit

The Complete Guide To Using Fitbit For Weight Loss and Increased Performance

RICHARD BOND

Copyright © 2015 Richard Bond

All rights reserved.

ISBN-13: 978-1515009726
ISBN-10: 1515009726

CONTENTS

INTRODUCTION

Dressing with new technologies is fashionable and certainly here to stay. Smart bracelets appear everywhere as an ultramodern accessory with a very interesting and futuristic technology footprint. They give that extra incentive for those who already practice or are thinking of starting a small or large range, unplanned, exercise. One can mainly interact with notifications on mobile and tablet or the measurement of information on exercise and health. They can become very interesting accessories for many independent users needing motivation.

When it comes to wearable devices, the first that comes to mind for many people is the famous Apple Smart Watch or else one of Smart Watches from Samsung, Motorola and LG. However, despite calling attention, these brands are far from the podium when the market is valued as a whole.

The concept of wearable technology is definitely here to stay and we have many indications of this. A recent report by ON World Institute predicted that 700 million wearable devices will be sold around the world over the next five years.

Although the idea of carrying a computer on the wrist seems strange to most people, the truth is that there are already several products available on international shelves that serve as an excellent gateway to this new category of gadgets. Smart bracelets - or smartbands, as they are being called - are an electronic increasingly common in the lives of many people, and can be very beneficial for organizing your daily life and boosting activity performance.

Within this segment, it is undeniable that the spotlights are centred on the Fitbit. The Fitbit Flex promises to monitor their user 24 hours a day obtaining various data, such as number of steps, distance, calories burned, hours slept and even the quality of their sleep. Clearly geared for those who like or want physical activities.

I've been a Fitbit user for some time now, and it took me some time to get the hang of its unique features. I checked on the main website and some other forums, but I learned most of what I know by experimenting with it. I've written this short guide to help the new Fitbit user. I am not sponsored by Fitbit, nor do I receive any commission for you choosing to buy their product. This is an honest assessment of my experience. There are some things I would change, which I'll come onto later, but overall I've been very pleased with it. I hope you in turn find some value from this guide, and make the most of this fitness tech.

WHAT DOES A FITBIT DO?

Some of you may already be aware of its features, while others might only know a fraction of its capabilities. In this chapter, I'm going to explore some of the main features of the watch.

Efficient user interface, but not always effective

The user interface Fitbit Flex is as simplistic as your own design. Different from Galaxy Gear Fit, for example, in that the bracelet does not have an LCD screen. Instead, it has five tiny LED lights that are used to communicate with the user.

When the user taps twice on the bracelet, a number of lights are illuminated relating to the percent completed of the established steps goal. Two LEDs lit means that 40% of the desired amount of daily steps has been reached. When you hit your target, Flex vibrates and lights up to congratulate the user. Five taps on the bracelet enters it into sleep mode, which is necessary every time you go to bed. From that moment, the Flex will now examine how much you move during the night, creating reports on the quality of your sleep. Two taps will just make a pair of LEDs light up quickly, remembering that you are in sleep mode.

Finally, to serve as an alarm clock, the bracelet also vibrates for a few seconds and lights a single LED to alert its user. If you do not dismiss the alarm (giving small touches on the device), it will enter a "snooze mode" and will activate again in nine minutes.

This interface based on small taps on the device is very simple and enjoyable, but it shows to be ineffective at times. During my the first few days of wearing it, my Flex entered sleep mode while I was riding my bike on a hilly terrain, misunderstanding the higher vibrations of the vehicle as human touches. I also found testimonies from other US users who had the same problem while driving cars using the bracelet. It's only happened a handful of times, but it's something to be mindful of.

A vast and open ecosystem

Like its mobile apps, the online panel of Fitbit is quite simple and easy to understand. It displays all data collected by Flex in a very organized way, separating different types of information blocks that can be arranged according to your need. The report is fairly complete, showing a history of activities done during the last few days, percentage of daily goal steps and minutes you spent doing heavy exercise. The sleep monitor shows how much you slept last night and how many times you woke during that period.

More than simply viewing data from your life, Fitbit panel also enables its users to manually enter some information that cannot be tracked by the gadget, such as calories consumed during meals and amount of water intake throughout the day.

However, this option cannot be fully utilized by users anywhere in the world, as the food database service has many snacks specific to North America. In addition, this feature is obviously catering to more attentive users about their own eating habits - after all, not everyone can say how many millimetres of water they drink daily.

One of the most interesting points of the Fitbit Flex in relation to their consumers is the fact that it is a "no frills bracelet," giving information as directly as possible. Unlike other smartbands available, the gadget has an open API that can be used by any developer interested in creating solutions that interact with the product. As a result, the Flex ecosystem is vast and growing, and you can connect your service with several other apps and websites that collects advanced data. Personally, I'm one for simplicity and efficiency, so this suits me perfectly.

MyFitnessPal, Microsoft HealthVault and MyFitLeague are just some of the many services that communicate with the intelligent Fitbit bracelet. I've been using the bracelet together with Endomondo (Windows Phone) and I can say that the combination works well. There's constant information exchanging between the two connected parts for you to utilize.

Even the IFTTT can be used in conjunction with your Fitbit: if you'd like to program it to publish a tweet profile when you reach 5000 steps, or send an SMS when the bracelet battery is running low. The possibilities are virtually endless: it all depends on your creativity and usage profile.

More than informing the weight, the recently launched scale Fitbit Aria Wi-Fi Smart Scale helps in motivation to achieve your goal. It feeds your profile on Fitbit to the site with data on the weight, the body fat percentage and BMI (Body Mass Index). This makes it possible to monitor and chart the evolution of fitness.

There are several models available and I'd like to touch on some of the key features of each one to help you make your decision:

Model One

• It is discreet, the silicone strap allows for use in the pocket, belt or underwear.

• Resistant to rain, splash and sweat.

• It has a monochrome OLED display. You can track your performance in real time, without the need for constant synchronization.

• Measurements are made with the use of accelerometer and high-precision altimeter.

• According to the manufacturer, it is the most accurate of similar devices.

• Monitors steps on stairs, distance and calories.

• The first line of Fitbit sleep monitor, via a strap placed overnight (hours, number of times awake, quality).

• Has a silent alarm that vibrates gently to wake the user.

• Battery life for seven days.

Model Zip

• Technology: Precision accelerometer.

• Has no altimeter.

• Resistant to rain, splash and sweat.

• LCD display. You can track your performance in real time, without the need to synchronize.

• Monitors number of steps, distance and calories.

• Has no sleep monitors.

• Does not monitor flights of stairs.

Flex Model

• Sleek and slim in bracelet form.

• Technology: Precision accelerometer.

• Has no altimeter.

• Resistant to rain, splash and sweat.

• Monitors number of steps, distance and calories.

• Monitor sleep (hours, number of times awake, quality).

• Does not monitor flights of stairs.

• Has a silent alarm that vibrates gently to wake the user.

• Various exchangeable bracelet colors.

• Precise Less than One model.

• Battery life for 10 days.

Model Force

• In wristband format, a bit thicker than the Flex model.

• Has hours on the display, which can replace the clock.

• It is the latest brand launch.

• Resistant to rain, splash and sweat.

• Contains lone button to change the display views.

• It has a blue OLED display. You can track your performance in real time, without the need for constant synchronization.

• Monitors steps of stairs, distance and calories.

• Monitors sleep (hours, number of times awake, quality).

• Technology: three-axis accelerometer and high-precision altimeter.

• Ready for IOS7 versions with functionality to notify you of incoming calls (vibrates and shows the name or number you are calling).

• Memory for 30 days.

• Battery life for 10 days.

• It is a direct competitor of Nike bracelet.

The table below shows some direct comparisons between the models:

	Force	Flex	One	Zip
Step Counter	•	•	•	•
Distance Travelled	•	•	•	•
Calories Burned	•	•	•	•
Stair Treads	•		•	
Goals Achieved	•	•		
Sleep Monitor	•	•	•	
Vibrating Alarm	•	•	•	

	Force	Flex	One	Zip
Syncs with Mac's and PC's	•	•	•	•
Syncs with Bluetooth 4.0*	•	•	•	•
Watch	•		•	•
Online Tools	•	•	•	•

The table below presents further comparisons between the models:

	Force	Flex	One	Zip
Display	OLED	LED	OLED	LCD
Estimated battery life	10 days	10 days	7 Days	6 months**
Battery types	Rechargeable	Rechargeable	Rechargeable	Rechargeable
Technology			Altimeter and Accelerometer	Accelerometer

Sync with Bluetooth devices: for mobile and IOS and Android tablets, this functionality requires the app (application), available only in the US.

Replaceable and non-rechargeable battery.

The use of technology for fitness can be a great alternative to break the monotony of the routine. The applications help to correlate and accelerate results. But care must be taken not to place all hope in these apparatuses, since the key to healthy weight loss is nutritional education combined with physical exercise and willpower. When used in the right way, fitness tech can become a great supplement to your training program.

Here are some other tools and apps that I've used and I would also recommend:

Smart Balance

More than informing the weight, the recently launched scale Fitbit Aria Wi-Fi Smart Scale helps motivate to achieve your goal. It feeds your profile on Fitbit with data on the weight of the site, the body fat percentage and BMI (Body Mass Index). This makes it possible to monitor and chart the evolution of weight loss and fitness. For those who want to avoid scares when stepping on the scale, Quantum can be a good option. The scale only tells you what you gained or lost since the last time you weighed, without revealing the total weight. This makes more evident the small achievements along the progression, since healthy weight loss happens gradually.

Diet and Health Application

The Diet and Health for iPhone app is the most downloaded app in the world, in the area of Health and Fitness. It is free and provides the nutritional information of over four thousand food (calories, carbohydrates, proteins, and fats). Also, send a current weight evaluation, ideal weight and BMI, and monitor the evolution in the weight loss process. Versions are available also for iPad and android.

Controlled physical activity

The BodyMedia Core Armband makes a report that counts burned calories, body temperature, and steps up duration and sleep efficiency as well as Fitbit while, being small, is practical to be used during running and other sports.

Video Game friend's diet

Games make the goal to lose weight more fun and are ideal for people who prefer physical activity indoors. There are exercises that mimic those carried out in gyms with weights and balls, or even options that blend traditional games with physical activity to burn more calories.

iPosture

A properly aligned spine is important to not let the most protruding belly look fatter. The iPosture is designed to send small vibrations every time that your posture is not correct, helping you to remember to correct it. An inch in diameter, it is practical for use under clothing all day.

My Fitness Pal

The application My Fitness Pal, available for Apple, BlackBerry, Windows Phone, and Android has many uses. Nutritionally, it helps to count the calories of meals and offers more than 600,000 suggestions for light recipes. In the exercises, it helps to compute physical activities. In addition, the application allows your friends on Twitter and Facebook help motivate you to continue the diet. Another similar application is the Noom Weight Loss, exclusive to Android, which uses GPS or pedometer to calculate the intensity of your workouts.

Exercises that fit in your pocket

The excuse of lack of money or laziness to exercise is no longer valid with the JEFIT application for Android and iPhone. The device has more than 300 exercises, all didactic and illustrated to help lose weight the healthy way. The application is indicated mainly to those who want to invest in weight training to lose fat and gain lean mass.

BENEFITS OF THE FEATURES

Fitbit Flex

The Flex allows you to monitor exercise activities during the day and when you are sleeping with wireless data synchronization for your computer, mobile phone, or tablet. Among the advantages are the possibility of putting a goal for a certain activity and the LED lights showing how you are doing. The bracelet can measure the number of steps taken, distance travelled, calories burned, active minutes, hours slept and even the quality of sleep.

A high-tech routine: After using the Fitbit Flex for several days, we can say that the bracelet achieves its goal of encouraging its members to lead a healthier life successfully. You may feel uncomfortable with the gadget on your arm during the first hours of use, but it's easy to get used to it after two or three days. Battery life on the Flex will last for about five days and recharges in two hours - to recharge, just plug it in the USB charger that came with the accessory.

Being water resistant, removing the bracelet even for bathing is not necessary - it is worth noting, however, that we observed the presence of some moisture inside the bracelet display after such an experience. Even though this water retained did no harm to the electronic device, it is nonetheless quite uncomfortable, which forced us to dry it out after putting it in the water.

You also need to get used to remember to enable and disable sleep mode at the correct times. Testing forgot to do this on two occasions, causing the Flex to register much longer naps and store data incompatible with reality. It would be interesting if the product was able to detect alone whenever you are actually sleeping, understanding the lack of movement as a period of well-deserved rest.

Immediate benefits guarantee incentive to work out, according to a study. Much more for those who think that exercise helps to improve the lives today, not the future. Experts in health and fitness have been trying for years to motivate people to exercise more using as arguments with a number of long-term benefits like losing weight, preventing heart disease, warding off dementia in old age and preventing the development of chronic diseases.

Sure, physical activity is actually good for everyone. But is the motivational message flawed from the beginning? New research shows that "improves heart health" can be much less effective an incentive message than, for example, "feel good now".

A study by the University of Michigan found that people are more likely to work out when the reasons are immediately applicable in their daily routine. For example, telling someone that she will have more energy after working out seems to be much better to say that exercising will make her less likely to develop diabetes.

For Michelle Segar, lead author of the study, the results indicate the need to improve the "propaganda" of the year. Just like that, she believes, the health organizations that promote physical activity in the summer get better results for their efforts.

We need to develop new messages that teach people that physical activity is one way to reduce stress, feel better, and have more energy at the time of activity and not only in the future. You become a more patient parent, perform better at work, and fight less with loved ones. The benefits of exercise can help you to lead a more enjoyable and productive life. That must be the message.

It been indicated that women valued long-term goals like weight loss, as much as short-term goals more directly linked to quality of life on a day-to-day basis, such as reducing stress. However, research found that women who cited short-term goals exercised more frequently than those considering long-term goals most important. People who exercised for quality of life were significantly more active than others.

Those who exercise based on the quality of daily life exercised 15% to 34% more, the study found. Specialists believe this finding points strongly to the need for reassessment of how exercise is promoted.

Health and healthy aging are very abstract concepts. We consider them important, but the problem lies in the fact that we live very busy, complicated lives. When you are looking at the list of your daily tasks, how attractive is it to fit a workout motivated by a reason that is in the distant future, that may not exist? If you are working out to improve the quality of your daily life, because the activity reduces stress and improves mood, you can see benefits immediately. And if you do not exercise, you will also feel worse immediately.

Messages of encouragement for people who need to exercise more frequently include: Feel better and thus become a more involved member of your family, improve productivity at work (working out makes the mind more focused), relieve the stress of everyday life, improve mood, enjoy higher energy levels and vitality in addition to having more time to enjoy social life itself and do outdoor activities.

Although these are quite compelling arguments for exercise, it is good to think twice before removing long-term goals to lead a better and healthier life. Long-term goals such as weight loss, tend to be measurable, while short-term goals - such as increased energy levels are largely subjective. The problem with the long-term goals is that people can work out for five and a half months and not lose a kilo. This is the case for short-term goals. Without a long-term goal, however, it is difficult to reach short-term goals.

Applications developed to help with training may be ideal for those who want guidance when it comes to working out. But before beginning any type of training, experts advise you undergo a medical exam to see if health conditions allow you to perform exercises. After all, even the low intensity training can pose risks to those who already have any kind of injury or chronic illness.

Also, for harder workouts, like those with weights or high performance racing, consulting a physical educator is very important. Small posture corrections, joint angles, intensity of charges and possible adjustments in training are essential for health.

Nike + Running

It is a very popular racing application. Allows running track, ability to share and compare your race anywhere and anytime, using the phone only. The GPS and accelerometer, e.g., record the distance, speed and training time with accuracy. It is also possible during the race, change the music and receive audio feedback to each kilometre run. To motivate the athlete, the application lets you share map path, the start of the race and the results on Facebook, as well as connect to nikeplus.com (a huge running group!). Free for iPhone and iPod Touch.

Runtastic

Works about the same as the previous one, allowing performance analysis through objective data for every workout. Also, it generates weekly and monthly statistics. The application includes a list of over 30 sports activities such as running, cycling, and skating, among others. For those who already run, it acts as a continuous stimulus, providing automatic tracking of distance, time, speed, pace, calories burned, altitude, heart rate, and other miscellaneous functions. Free for iPhone and Android.

Sports Tracker

Great for those who enjoy cycling, walking, running and other physical activity based on distance. It allows you to create diagrams and personalized training plans. In addition to maps, it offers calculation of time and distance travelled, step counter, calories burned and altitude from training and races. Associated with a compatible monitor also measures the heart rate. Finally, the program share data, photos and music heard on the application site and on Facebook. Free for iPhone.

Cyclist Pro GPS +

Allows the experience of pedalling to be quantified, giving the user the ability to determine how far you want to go or how many calories you want to burn. It also shows speed, distance, generates maps and reports for optimal monitoring.

GAIN Fitness

Creates individualized exercise, based on knowledge of professional trainers certified. It has over 700 activities (resistance, plyometric training, yoga, etc.) and can create others, tailored to you. The app also has easy tracking and monitoring activities. Then sync with the site allows the user to manage their training online or by phone. Free for iPhone.

Endomondo

Manages time, distance, speed and calories burned. Ideal for those who practice sports such as cycling, running or walking. The app synchronizes all activities with a website and provides the path on Google Maps, in addition to sharing information on Facebook and Twitter. Free for iPhone, Android and BlackBerry.

FITBIT FUN

The social factor has not been forgotten by Fitbit. If you know someone who also uses the bracelet, you can add them to your list of friends and compete to see who takes the longest walks in a given time interval. This system may seem somewhat "rough" for those watching from a distance, but believe me: the simple fact of knowing that there is a computer analyzing everything you do and that there is a daily goal waiting to be fulfilled is enough to encourage you to use more legs and less car.

Wireless communication with any device

The Fitbit Flex is a wireless bracelet - that is, all communication with your computer or mobile device is done by wireless means. It uses the Bluetooth 4.0 technology to transfer data, which consumes much less power than previous versions of such communication protocol.

The process to activate it is quite simple. With the bracelet properly "dressed", all you need to do is connect a small USB dongle (included with the device) into your computer and open the synchronization software that can be found on the manufacturer's website. Then simply create an account with the service and wait for the first match between the software and the wearable device. In less than five minutes my Flex was already properly configured.

The process to sync it to tablets and smartphones is the same. The official Fitbit app download for your gadget (there is a version for iPhone and one for Android, Windows Phone is coming soon) and perform the pairing. From the time when the flex is synchronized with given computer or mobile device, the data exchange is performed automatically every 20 minutes - obviously, the USB dongle must be connected to the machine and the Bluetooth tablet or cell in question must always be on.

Engaging in friendly competitions with friends, family, or work colleagues can keep you motivated to lose weight. Some people may find that peer pressure in a competition helps them improve health, get proper nutrition and exercise regularly. A weight loss challenge is also a good way to form a support network for those involved so that they can maintain their new lifestyle when the challenge ends.

Find people willing to participate. Look around your community and network of friends to determine who might be willing to hold a weight loss challenge. If you prefer not to directly approach people, publish a notice so people know how to contact you if they are interested. For example, ask your pastor if you can put a note in the church bulletin about the idea of a weight loss challenge. You can also do the same in a publication at work.

Determine the nature of the weight loss challenge. For example, you can launch a competitive challenge in which participants stay lean as much as you can within a period of time. Alternatively, you can create a non-competitive challenge in which each individual is encouraged to fulfil a personal weight loss goal. In any of these scenarios, you may have regular weight measurements throughout the challenge to allow people to monitor their progress. Those who are losing weight are congratulated and those that do not receive support and encouragement.

Establish a schedule for the challenge. If you want to create a number of challenges, set a schedule for each, which allows people to enter the routine of weight loss and create a total change of lifestyle so that new healthy habits remain. For example, you may want to launch a new challenge every three months with weekly checks.

Decide whether the challenge will be semi-private or public. Decide whether any progress will be made available to all participants, or if only the "winner" of each week will be revealed. If a participant does not want their particular results revealed weekly, their privacy should be respected in order to maintain the project's friendly atmosphere.

Establish a database to monitor the statistics of the challenge and choose one or two trusted people to keep them confidential. Alternatively, you may wish to have participants self-report their progress each week to administrators and also have participants self-report their result at the end of the challenge.

Decide on the prize or reward at the end of the challenge. Participants can donate money to buy prizes or your company may want to sponsor you if the challenge is in a workplace. If your challenge is large enough, local businesses may be willing to donate a prize for the winner or who reaches the goal. Awards to participate must also be considered for people who signed up for the challenge and stayed until the end.

Plan and execute motivational events and activities to encourage healthy eating and exercise. For example, if a participant is an amateur chef, she can stand ready to provide a healthy cooking class to help participants plan meals. If a participant is an outdoor activity enthusiast, he may be willing to lead a local walk. Keep the fun and low pressure activities for people to want to participate.

Devices that count calories from food, regulate the level and efficiency of physical activities and to control body posture. The use of technology for fitness can be a great alternative to break the monotony of the routine. Experts in Nutrition Functional Clinical applications help to quantify and still accelerate results. "But we must be careful not to place all hope in these devices as the key to a healthy weight loss is food combined rehabilitation with physical exercise and willpower".

GOALS & THE IMPORTANCE OF PUTTING THE WORK IN

Why is it so difficult to overcome laziness and inertia to start practicing physical activities? "Human nature has a tendency to repeat old habits and to resist the new," explains behavioral psychologist. What to do then? "It takes at least six months for a new routine turn a consolidated habit. Meanwhile we must persist, even unwilling," says sports psychologist. Deep down, we know that, right? But do not be discouraged. You do not need to think about the failures when trying to incorporate physical activity into your daily life. I will go through ten tricks that worked very well with me to make your mind work to your advantage in the battle against inactivity.

If you are just starting a training program you must start slowly and increase the intensity and the level of exercise gradually. Some people almost die on the first day of training; they get hurt or get extremely sore muscles and joints (or both) and end up abandoning workouts at the gym or outdoors. If you are a sedentary person, start with 15-20 minute walk in the first two weeks and then increase the intensity and add weight training. Be smart and start slowly!

Something very common in the gym is to see lost people, not knowing what to do or how to use the machines. This will over time discouraging the person and so many people just disappearing from the gym after a month. Look for books, e-books, magazines, websites, and blogs where you can learn how to use the gym and get faster results. Hiring a personal trainer is a great alternative for you to learn what to do to succeed in your goals. Never stop learning and change your training routine every 4 weeks.

Let the gym be your priority in your daily routine. Plan to go work out in a time that is always specific and convenient for your day-to-day or you will "push" the gym for later and just never go.

Look for a training companion! Training with a partner is much more fun and you end up encouraging and motivating each other to give their best during training. The training ends up being a compromise and the days when you think about not going, you end up going because he knows that is committed to their partnership. One important thing: within the gym the conversation you should be ONLY about fitness! Let other conversations wait for after training, so you do not lose the focus and intensity of the workout!

Goal setting is more important than you may think. If you do not where to go, you will not know how to get there! Plan REAL goals for yourself both long and short term. Every time you achieve one of your goals get yourself a reward for your efforts.

Tips

- Keep a diary: Register your goals and your progress in physical activities in a daily paper, on a blog or social networks. Sharing your goals helps you not give them up and gives motivation in difficult times.

- Be inspired by someone: Stick on the fridge a full body picture of a woman or man you want to look like or even a picture of your past. Say to yourself, as often as necessary, "I will achieve this, or even better!"

- Start slowly: At the beginning of exercise, your body will be sore. A little pain will soon pass, but it may be enough to discourage.

- Choose an exercise that has already given you positive experiences in the past, that you enjoy doing.

- Start with the most basic class and then increase the difficulty only when you realize that the level at which it is now easy for you;

- Create realistic goals: Weight loss of 30 kg or having the flat belly of a super elite athlete are impossible short term goals. Keep the long-term goal in mind, but create more immediate goals, such as eliminating 1 kg or 1 cm of belly in a few weeks.

- <u>Earn rewards</u>: Establish a presence in the classroom or in training as a weekly goal, and give yourself a reward if you fulfil it. After each surpassed goal, establish a prize (other than food). It may be a new outfit, a perfume, a walk, or something will motivate you enough to continue pursuing your goals. Everyone needs motivation. Share your goals with people you know who will be rooting for you. They will be your support in times of discouragement.

- <u>Fit exercise into your routine</u>: It is easier to acquire a new habit when it fits into their daily lives. If you are going into a gym, choose one near your home or work. Determine fixed days and times for exercise, the activity needs to take time and some space in your life.

- <u>Have "reference pants"</u>: Register your evolution, every day check and record your score for your perceived exertion and build a picture of your changes. If you want to lose weight or trim your waist, prove it to yourself every week by wearing the same pants. It is easier to notice small changes in your body like this rather than looking in the mirror.

- <u>Work out soon</u>: Choose an environment where you feel comfortable to exercise. If you do not like the people in your gym, try another. There are dozens of options besides treadmill, bike and weights: dance lessons, hiking, martial arts, yoga, water aerobics, capoeira, team sports, etc. But if after two weeks it remains a burden, it's time to switch to something more fun. The important thing is to feel good.

- <u>Search for a companion</u>: In the company of someone you care about, exercise time passes faster and you have more encouragement to continue. If you have no company, make friends at the gym.

- <u>Stop sabotaging</u>: Set goals in the medium and long term, describe what you need to do to achieve them and what will be the reward later. Include fun in physical activity, inviting people close to your level, or preferably already more advanced than you to train with you and listening to the songs you like. Often if you fail to exercise in a day, you'll give up doing the next also. Thoughts like "it's no big deal if I break this promise" followed by a sense of failure are typical of sabotage acts. If you fail to do the exercise one day, and resume straight away!

TIPS & TRICKS

I'd like to share some tips and tricks that might assist your health and well-being goals that you can use alongside your Fitbit.

Turning life into a challenging game

In short, the intelligent Fitbit bracelet has five distinct features. It tracks your steps, distance travelled, calories burned, sleep quality and also acts as an alternative alarm clock, vibrating softly on the user's pulse on a predetermined schedule. Unfortunately, the model does not have an altimeter to record flights of stairs you climb or descend. All this collected data is stored locally within a maximum period of seven days - meaning, if you do not synchronize your Flex for a week, any old information will automatically be erased and will be impossible to get it back.

More than simply counting how many steps you took last Saturday, the gadget also serves as an incentive for a healthier life by applying the concept of gamification to their screening system. You can determine a personal daily goal of steps you need to walk to keep fit - by default, this goal is 10,000 steps per day. As you exercise, the Flex will congratulate you by offering collectable virtual medals in a system that closely resembles the Achievements found in video games.

How about making money to work out? Changing a bad habit is not a simple task. In fact, some would say it is impossible. The same is true when it comes to acquiring a good habit. However beneficial it can be to exercise and eat healthy foods, the vast majority of people succumb to laziness, troubled routines and fatty foods. You cannot exterminate a behaviour once it is a habit, but you can replace a bad or evil habit for a more positive behavior. It is important to note that feelings or situations lead us to repeat certain negative action and then to put this action into practice, regardless of the reward. If you are able to identify the actions and rewards, you can change the habit.

But to do all of this alone sounds both tedious and complicated. Technology, however, can already help. The three applications described below encourage people to eat well and maintain an exercise routine. No, they do not just pass you a packed menu of fruits and vegetables or a miraculous series of sit-ups and jogging on the treadmill. What they do is move in a somewhat gentler place: your pocket. Like a reward for walking in line, applications offer users money. Don't believe it? Check it out.

Diet Bet

This application works with two challenging levels. The first, Kickstarter, has four weeks and the goal is that you lose 4% of your body weight. Then, the Transformer diet lasts one to four months and the objective is to reduce weight by 10%. Participants can interact and share their good results via a platform on Facebook and the app, and receive advice and support. Once the registration is carried out in the application, the user pays a certain amount in a Pay Pal account or credit card. If you meet your goal, you get back your deposit plus more money from those that did not meet the goals shared by all the winners. Mindful of the wise guys, the application prompts the user to upload two photos as soon as the game starts: a full-length on a scale and more, closely, to show their initial weight. Over time, the "Player" is weighed and uploads new photos. To prevent cheating, the application sends keywords that should be placed on the floor next to the scale at the time the photo.

Wage Healthy

You fill in how much you want to lose and calculate how much you can win. Then you can decide on how long you plan to take to achieve your goal and how much you're willing to bet on it per month. From then you control what you eat, exercising and not giving up. Prizes can be quite attractive. For example, for someone who wants to lose 12 kilos in six months and bet $50 per month, reaching their challenge, you can earn between US $500 and US $1,230.

Entries in the application can be done in three ways: individually, collectively (with the creation of a team of five people, whether friends, colleagues, or family) and also a second form of collective game: with the staff at work. The company you work for can sign up in the game and ask employees to participate in the challenge. To deposit and receive money, you must use a credit card or PayPal account.

Gym Pact

In this application, the user takes weeks with goals to eat well and / or work out. If you do not meet your goals, you will be penalized and will pay an amount to be divided among the participants who have achieved their goals. Among the agreements that can be made are eating 15 servings of vegetables a week, running five times or write a food diary regularly . Every pact requires at least a bet of $5, but you can increase this value to feel more motivated (and more afraid of losing money). The rewards are not as good as the other applications, but the incentive to not lose money can be quite useful for those who want to change their eating and exercise habits.

These three applications will not make you rich, but can help you become a healthier and disciplined person. Who knows, with new habits will your chances of being more focused at work be greater? And who knows, might you be rewarded for it with a promotion or pay raise?

The Fitbit Aria scale is smart to measure your weight, body fat percentage and BMI (body mass index) to provide an overview of weight. This scale helps you reach your weight goals, allowing you to set goals, track your progress effortlessly and stay motivated every day. Your stats automatically carry through its Wi-Fi panel, where you can get a more comprehensive view of your health and fitness, and track your eating and exercise habits. The scale can be configured to automatically recognize up to 8 users. You can check your progress from your computer or with a free smartphone application.

MY FITBIT SUMMARY

The usefulness of Fitbit Flex depends largely on your user profile. If you're looking for a bracelet whose primary function is to act as an extension of your mobile phone - sending notifications and running simple applications, such as the Razer Nabu and Gear Fit - Flex was definitely not made for you. As made explicit in this analysis, the product is somewhat simplistic in its communication with the user and acts discreetly on your wrist, limited only to track information, and not display it.

On the other hand, if you are a person who practices frequent walks and strives to lead a healthy life, the product shows to be an amazing gadget to automate your routine in a magical way. It also serves as a nice incentive to start a fitness routine, since it is impossible not to feel motivated to hit your goals daily, unlock achievements and compete against your friends through the online service panel.

Personally speaking, I myself walk much more than usual, having developed certain anticipation to see the five Flex LED lights congratulating me for meeting the 10 000 steps to the end of each day: a sense of accomplishment is rewarding and it pays off.

The Fitbit Flex design divides opinions - some consider it an accessory with a minimalist and understated look, perfect to use without attracting the attention of potential thieves. On the other hand, there are those who compare the bracelet with children's watches made of cheap plastic. I personally quite like the look of the device, and I'm more in line with the first group mentioned. Although it is not as attractive as the Jawbone UP, the Flex appeals by adopting a simplistic concept and follow the trend of "more is less".

It is worth noting that the unit itself comes down to a tiny module that can be easily removed from inside the bracelet - the plastic strap can be changed according to the user's will, and you can find it in several different colors and sizes (being the gadget box comes with a bracelet in small size and one full size).

The versatility of Flex opens interesting possibilities; as recently reported, the luxury label Tory Burch announced a beautiful gold plated bracelet for those who want to turn your device into a true "electronic gem". Not for me personally, but for some looks are important.

If these are the features that you expect from a smart band do not hesitate to buy a Fitbit Flex - and if possible, try to do it outside the country, for the price it's not an appropriate value for the resources that the bracelet has the offer. In the international market they are perfectly consistent with the strengths and weaknesses of the device and you can even see the lack of an altimeter.

In fact, using a Flex is an excellent way to enter the world of wearable devices. This market has yet to show its real power, but a fairly cheap and simple gadget like this, the Fitbit has an important role start getting used to the idea of having a computer watching us intimately during day and night, turning into another electronic accompanying us everywhere we go.

I hope you've found this guide useful and informative, and in some way has helped you make the most of your watch, or at least your decision to buy one or not.

Whatever you decide to do, I wish you the best of luck with your health and well-being goals.

OTHER BOOKS BY RICHARD BOND

Your First Marathon – A Beginners Guide To Marathon Training, Marathon Preparation And Completing Your First Marathon

Your First Triathlon – A Beginners Guide To Triathlon Training, Triathlon Preparation And Completing Your First Triathlon

Mental Toughness - A Guide to Developing Peak Performance and an Unbeatable Mind in Everyday Life

www.ingramcontent.com/pod-product-compliance
Lightning Source LLC
Chambersburg PA
CBHW060347290526
45791CB00004B/1576